Anti-Inflammatory Swaps Made Easy-ish

An easy-ish guide to managing inflammation

MARQUITA VALENTINE

Dedication

To my family, I love each of you so much. I am so proud of the way we came together to support one another during this season of our lives. Team W, all the way.

Contents

Disclaimer

This publisher and author disclaim liability for any medical outcomes that may occur as a result of applying the methods suggested in this book. In other words, consult your doctor or another health-trained professional FIRST.

The information contained in this guide is not a substitute for professional medical advice or medical treatment. I am only sharing what has worked and continues to work for all members of our family, but especially for our youngest, who has pediatric Crohn's Disease. We continuously work with a pediatric Crohn's specialist and a functional nutritionist, who is also a licensed medical doctor, to monitor our son's health. Please consult your doctor and/or a specialist to see if an anti-inflammatory diet might work for you or your loved one.

Dear Reader,

In the fall of 2022, our youngest—a healthy, active, 15-year-old varsity soccer player—suddenly became ill. Within six weeks, he lost twenty-five pounds, could barely keep any food in him, had little to no energy, wasn't interested in eating, and every specialist who saw him had a different yet still incorrect diagnosis.

To say that we were worried is an understatement. I don't think my husband and I have ever felt as powerless as we did during this time, as we searched for answers, had what felt like every test on Earth performed on our son, and he remained sick. Barely eating and incredibly tired, it was hard for him to go to school each day. This kid, who loved to eat, hang out with friends, and play soccer, was no longer interested in any of those things.

And this is the part where I can't stress enough how important it is for you or someone you trust to advocate either for you, your child, your spouse, your relative, your friend … whoever you love who is not getting the answers they need to heal.

On December 31st, 2022, we reached our breaking point. After a fun family night, our youngest spiked a fever of 103.6, and it wouldn't come down, no matter what we did, so my husband drove our son to the emergency room and said he wasn't leaving until he got answers.

Now, I have to tell you, my 6'4 husband, while confident and sure of himself, is not the type to throw his weight (or height) around for the heck of it or even yell. He's the calm one in our relationship, but we were way past the calm or even the waiting stage. We needed definitive answers with definitive solutions.

Finally, nearly three months after our son's initial illness, we had an answer—pediatric Crohn's Disease. I'd like to say that this made things easier; that we were like, oh, cool, well, let's get to curing this thing. But that didn't exactly happen. For one, we were in total shock. We thought for sure it was some kind of virus or bacterial infection. Second, neither of us knew very much, if anything, about Crohn's, and we especially had no idea that there wasn't (and still isn't) a cure and that it wasn't common in kids. Although, it is increasing, just like all chronic diseases in kids, much to the befuddlement of many specialists and other doctors.

As of right now, the specialists we've spoken to do not know if Crohn's Disease is caused by genetics or something else that triggers it, or a combination of the two. It's one of life's mysteries that hasn't been solved … yet.

BUT GOD! (Hallelujah and Amen) During that time of uncertainty, I was listening to my favorite podcasts like The Office Ladies, Allie Beth Stuckey's Relatable, and Alex

Clark's The Spillover, which is now Culture Apothecary, for all different reasons, but mainly because I wanted the distraction from the never-ending anxiety and weird parent guilt that I was somehow responsible for my genetics that I may or may not have passed on to our son, and reality of being helpless as anything.

Through two of those podcasts, I learned about anti-inflammatory foods, products, and so-called alternatives—medical therapies that didn't involve pharmaceuticals or used a combination of diet, aka food, and pharmaceutical therapies.

Guest after guest talked about inflammation and its effect on our bodies, regardless of any medical diagnosis. It was all about what you put in your body, being what you'll get out, and educating oneself on what's in our food (good and bad). As a former teacher, I absolutely loved that suggestion.

So, by the time we got the diagnosis, it was easy-peasy, and we were totally prepared. Narrator: It was, in fact, NOT easy-peasy, and they were totally unprepared.

Our son was given steroids to get his appetite back and to calm the inflammation. Meanwhile, we had to decide if we were going to use pharmaceutical therapies to "get" our son in remission. Our specialists reviewed the pros and cons, including the side effects, with us, which take a massive toll on the body, especially a child's body. Solely because of the podcast episodes that I'd been listening to and sharing with my husband, we asked about using food. Thankfully, that was an option that our specialists were open to trying.

*(Disclaimer: If our son needed immediate intervention via surgery or chemotherapy-type transfusions, we would've agreed to whatever he needed to get healthy *while* eating an anti-inflammatory diet.)*

Overwhelmed by all the information we'd been given by the hospitals' nutritionists, books on Crohn's Disease and inflammation, and podcasts that talked about any of the above, my husband and I decided to work with a functional nutritionist to get the best of both worlds, and our specialist completely supported our decision. In fact, I'd say that the two of them are among the best doctors we've ever worked with due to their genuine concern for our son, unhurried manner, and active listening skills.

*What resulted from that was my husband, and I decided that our entire family would go on the same anti-inflammatory diet as our youngest so that he could be successful and feel supported. This meant that our whole lifestyle changed, from the cleaning products we used to the food we ate, to our water, and even to how or if we could eat at *any* restaurants.*

This also meant spending hours in the grocery store reading labels for weeks on end and looking up what the ingredients consisted of—not because all chemicals / ingredients were unhealthy per se—but rather because certain ingredients were known to be inflammatory for someone with Crohn's Disease.

After six months, I was able to get my weekly grocery shopping down to an hour or less, but I realized other families don't have schedules like mine, or other families of all kinds are exhausted once they finally have a break in their schedule, and the last thing they want to do is spend hours in the grocery store.

That's where this guide comes in.

I've already done the work, read the ingredients, sampled the products, modified the recipes, and I have the time to continue to do this.

My goal is to share this with you, Dear Reader, so that you can make informed decisions on what's best for your family without spending untold hours at the grocery store or online (I read a lot of labels there, too!).

In this book, you will see that I recommend organic, non-GMO products, produce, meat, etc., but if you absolutely can't afford the grocery bill that goes along with that (believe me, we know, but it's still cheaper than what we would have to pay in medical treatments), don't stress. I will give you a list of what can give you the most benefit for your money, and then you can decide what to do with the rest of your groceries and other swaps. There is no shame in doing what you can, and there is no shame in slowly changing / swapping out the old with the new.

To date, our son is still in remission, without pharmaceutical therapies, and is a healthy 6'2 seventeen-year-old. Personally, my migraines are now dependent on the weather instead of the food I eat. My husband had the best physical this year (it was so good his doctor, who was previously concerned about the diet we were following, asked him to share more in-depth information about it with him). Our oldest says she can tell an immense difference between what she eats at home and what she eats when out with friends and during the year while she's living on campus.

If you have any questions and would like to sign up for my newsletter (I also write sweet romance and am revamping all of my previously deleted social media accounts to reflect this change.) to receive updates, sales information, and recipes, please email me at marquita@marquita valentine.com. You can find me on Facebook and Instagram, too.

-Marquita

Anti-inflammatory Food Swaps

- Look for labels that say non-GMO, organic, and, when possible (although harder to find), regenerative farming practices.

- Avoid corn syrup, soy, corn, most kinds of wheat, vegetable oil, cottonseed oil, canola oil, corn oil, rapeseed oil, grapeseed oil, soybean oil, sunflower oil, sesame oil, natural flavors, artificial dyes, high sugar / sucrose, A1 dairy, most legumes, and most peanuts.

- Read the ingredient list on every label. Don't ever be afraid to email a company to ask for clarification, or if they would be willing to swap out an inflammatory ingredient for a less inflammatory one.

- Our diet is protein-heavy and works for us. A plant-based diet would require our son's body to do too much work to break down the plants used in vegan diets, so if you're looking for a plant-based or plant-heavy diet, this is not the guide for you.

- Support small farmers and buy locally whenever possible.

Little Things Made Easy-ish

Before you read through this guide, I want to highlight some of the little things we do to help our son stay in remission because they really add up to equal big results. Also, I say diet a lot, but it doesn't mean what we 80s/90s babies were taught—it just means a type of food plan we follow, not a calorie-deficit plan.

We don't eat the skins of apples, grapes, legumes, or potatoes. Normally, this would be encouraged to help with fiber intake and nutrients. Unfortunately, for our son, this is extra fiber his body does not need, nor does he need his body to work harder to break it down. That's also why we do not eat vegetables like broccoli and broccolini.

Chew your food! Digestion starts in the mouth, but we have been trained to eat quickly (I say this as a former classroom teacher, so it's part of the school day as well to hurry up and eat!). We need to retrain and reclaim our time to enjoy food and each other's company while eating.

You don't have to do everything all at once. Little steps add up to make giant leaps forward. Personally, I found it very stressful at first because I wanted to change everything all at once, and it just wasn't humanly possible. Instead, focus on what you can change to make your body less inflammatory.

In fact, I start with the top three things you can change to get the biggest results for the least amount of money. However, if you can only afford to change one thing—then make it your mission to be seed oil free. You will see the most significant results by removing canola, vegetable, grapeseed, cottonseed, and soybean oil from your food, including when you cook.

The Big Three Swaps Made Easy-ish!

All oils, sugars, and flours are not created the same.

This is where you'll get the best results from an anti-inflammatory swap, and it's by swapping out the three things that we all use the most.

Cooking / Baking Oils

- Coconut Oil (Carrington Farms)
- Avocado Oil (Chosen Brand)
- Olive Oil (California Olive Ranch – 100% California label)
- Animal fat / tallow

Flours

- Bob's Red Mill Super Fine Almond Flour
- King Arthur's 1 to 1 GF Flour
- Jovial's All Purpose Einkorn Flour (wheat-based)
- Viddie's Bakery Ultra Fine White Rice Flour

Sweeteners (Use Sparingly)

- Raw sugar
- Honey
- Maple Syrup
- Powdered Sugar
- Brown Sugar
- Stevia

Seasonings / Herbs

Seasonings can not only enhance and bring out the flavor of good food, but they can also aid in digestion and lower inflammation in our bodies. Our go-to's: turmeric, paprika, pepper, salt, garlic powder, cayenne pepper, and onion powder.

- Turmeric
- Ginger
- Cinnamon
- Ground Mustard
- Oregano
- Cayenne Pepper
- Garlic
- Garlic Salt
- Onion Powder
- Rosemary
- Salt
- Kosher Salt

- Black Ground Pepper
- Paprika
- Thyme
- Cumin
- Dill
- Siete Taco Seasoning
- Old Bay
- Tarragon
- Curry
- Saffron
- Pluck Seasonings

Condiments / Sauces / Additions

This category was super easy for our youngest since he doesn't eat ketchup, mayonnaise, mustard, or other condiments. His "plain" eating made it easier for him to change how he eats. But don't worry; the rest of us eat those things, so I scouted out the best ones.

- Heinz Simple Ketchup (uses cane sugar *but* also has natural flavors—our son doesn't eat ketchup, and I don't use this as an addition to anything I make. However, this is my favorite ketchup, and is in that 10% of the time I'm not eating totally inflammatory free.)
- Primal Kitchen Ketchup (no sugar and your best choice)
- Mustard (use an organic, no artificial dyes or flavor brand)
- Chosen Mayonnaise
- Pickles (no artificial dyes)

- Coconut Secret Liquid Coconut Aminos (our version of soy sauce)
- Tomato Sauce / Paste (use a brand that is non-GMO and contains only tomatoes, or tomatoes and water as ingredients)

Easy-ish Ranch Dressing / Dip Recipe

½ cup of sour cream

½ cup of mayonnaise

½ tsp of salt

¾ tsp of pepper

½ tsp of garlic powder

½ tsp of onion powder

1-2 tablespoons of dill weed

Directions:

- Combine all wet and dry ingredients into a bowl and whisk together. Add water if necessary for the thickness of a salad dressing.

Protein Powders & Fiber

- Be Well By Kelly – any flavor without peanut butter
- Taylor Dukes Wellness Bone Broth
- Anthony's Organic Acacia Powder
- Truvani (plant-based)

Nut Butters

- Barney's Almond Butter (no salt, no sugar added, does use palm oil)
- Valencia Peanuts Peanut Butter
- Any organic nut butter with bare minimum ingredients (no sugar added)

Easy-ish Protein Shake Recipe

1 scoop of your favorite protein powder

1-2 tablespoons of preferred nut butter

1-2 tablespoons of acacia powder

½ cup of ice (optional; I enjoy mine milkshake thick)

1 banana (optional; only my husband adds it to his)

1 ½ cups of almond milk

Directions:

- Add all ingredients to your blender and blend to the desired consistency.

12

Bread

- Canyon Bakehouse GF Bread / Bagels
- Cristal Burger Buns and Sub Rolls
- Make your own with a bread machine

Butter

- Truly Butter
- Challenge Butter
- Kerry Gold Butter
- Vital Farms Butter (avocado oil)
- Vital Farms Ghee
- Make your own

Easy-ish Butter Recipe

2 cups of heavy cream

One kitchen aid blender, hand mixer, or food processor

Cheesecloth

Directions:

- Pour 2 cups of heavy cream into a bowl
- Blend until the butter separates
- Scoop butter onto cheesecloth, cover, and rinse under cold water, then squeeze out excess until water runs clear.
- Add salt, honey, or herbs.

Dairy

- A2 Cow's Milk
- Raw Milk
- A2 Heavy cream (no lactose)
- Almond Milk (Elmhurst Brand only has two ingredients)
- Green Valley Lactose-Free Sour Cream
- Alec's A2 Ice Cream
- Cosmic Bliss plant-based Ice Cream (coconut-based but no coconut taste)
- A2 Cow's Milk Yogurt
- Goat's Milk Yogurt
- Coconut Milk Based Yogurt
- LaClare Goat's Cheese—mozzarella, raw cheddar
- Any aged, hard cheese
- Green Valley Lactose-Free Cream Cheese

Easy-ish Bagel Recipe

- 1 cup of gluten-free or Einkorn flour
- 1 cup yogurt of choice
- 1 tsp baking soda (optional)
- 1 tsp baking powder (optional)
- 1 tsp salt (optional)

Directions:

- Preheat Oven to 375
- Add all ingredients into a mixing bowl, and then combine until a sticky and slightly crumbly dough is formed.
- Dump out onto a lightly floured surface and roll out a couple of times, then separate into four large balls or six medium balls.
- Form into bagel shapes and place on a baking pan lined with parchment paper.
- Bake for 15-18 minutes.

Potato Chips and Corn Alternative Nacho Chips

- Boulder Canyon Chips (uses avocado oil)
- Siete Chips
- Siete "Tortilla" Chips (cassava based)
- Vandy's Chips (uses beef tallow)
- The Good Crisp Company (their version of Pringles is chef's kiss!)

Easy-ish Chip Recipe

Russet potatoes (1-2 per person)
Refined Coconut Oil (2 cups melted in a large saucepan)
Sea Salt to desired taste

Directions:
- Cut into thin slices.
- Fry in coconut oil until crispy, then remove and place on a plate covered with a paper towel to absorb excess oil.
- Transfer to bowl and toss with sea salt.
- Store in an airtight container.

Snacks

With all this talk of healthier eating, you might be shocked or at least surprised that I included a snack category, but like I said, this isn't a diet where we stop eating entire categories of food unless they contain seed oils, dyes, etc.

Everyone, especially kids, loves to have snacks and drinks after school / work or in their lunchboxes, and they don't want to be left out of events or parties (or holidays). So, I've rounded up our favorite snacks and baked goods that meet our dietary restrictions while tasting delicious.

- Surf Sweets and Yum Earth (candy and gummy bears / worms)
- Simple Mills Brand for snacks and to bake at home (some of their products use sunflower oil)
- Siete Brand cookies and churro strips
- Choco Yums (an M&M's alternative)
- Lesser Evil Popcorn (our daughter's favorite)

- Jovial Sourdough Crackers

- Bob's Red Mill Brand – for cookies and brownies to make at home

- Make your own popcorn; just make sure the corn is non-GMO and organic (This is something our son eats rarely.)

Drinks

- Apple Juice (Apple and Eve)
- White Grape Juice
- Lemonade (organic brand with no natural flavors added, lemons, water, and sugar only) or make your own
- Sweet or Unsweet Tea—organic and doesn't contain microplastics
- Filtered Water
- Olipop (carbonated, flavored tonic with good ingredients)

Beef, Chicken, and Seafood

- Beef (Good Ranchers Subscription or buy local)
- Chicken (Good Ranchers Subscription or buy local)
- Whole Chicken (Springer Mountain Farms or buy local)
- Salmon (Make sure whatever brand of seafood you buy is wild caught—not farmed—in the USA)
- Shrimp
- Flounder
- Sea Bass
- Cod
- Canned Tuna – Safe Catch Brand (tests for mercury levels)
- Turkey Breast
- Deli meat—Make your own, or buy a brand that uses only salt, water, potato starch, and the actual meat.
- Despite our southern heritage and Eastern North Carolina BBQ sauce recipe, which has been passed down through the generations, we no longer eat pork.

Easy-ish Crab or Tuna Cake Recipes

2 cans of crab or tuna

½ c of mayonnaise

1 egg

2 tablespoons of coconut aminos

½ cup of almond flour

½ cup of milk (your choice)

½ tsp of salt

½ tsp of pepper

1 tablespoon of Old Bay Seasoning

Directions:

- Preheat Oven to 375

- Mix all ingredients together. They should be able to form a slightly loose "cake". If they're too liquidy, add more almond flour. If too dense, add more milk.

- Spoon onto a baking pan lined with parchment paper, or use a large muffin pan with cupcake liners.

- Sprinkle more Old Bay Seasoning on top.

- Bake for about 25 minutes.

Vegetables / Legumes / Rice / Tubers / Noodles

- Carrots (always peel)
- Sweet Potatoes
- Russet or Gold Potatoes (always peel or don't eat skin for baked potato)
- Green Beans
- Squash
- Bok Choy
- Spinach
- Collards
- Lettuce (use sparingly)
- Micro Greens
- Tomatoes
- Celery (to cook with, not eat raw or cooked)
- Onions
- Bell Peppers
- Black beans (eat with rice)
- Mushrooms

- Cucumbers
- Beets
- Jovial GF Noodles
- 4Sisters White Rice

Easy-ish Rice Recipe

1 cup of rice

2 cups of water or chicken broth

Rice Maker

Add ingredients to rice maker, close lid, and press white rice or brown rice. It's done when it sings or beeps.

Fruits

- Cantaloupe
- Pineapple
- Apples (always peeled)
- Blueberries
- Strawberries
- Bananas
- Pears
- Avocado
- Mangoes
- Watermelon
- Peeled Grapes (seedless)
- Oranges
- Lemons
- Limes
- Avocadoes
- Pomegranates
- Figs
- Dates

Easy-ish Fruit Side Dish

Combine the following into a bowl:

½ of a watermelon, diced

½ cup of thinly sliced red onions

2-3 tablespoons of lime juice

salt and pepper to taste

Optional: add goat's cheese.

Baking

- Apple Cider Vinegar (make sure the brand isn't using APEEL apples)
- Anthony's Active Yeast Packets
- Baking Powder
- Baking Soda
- Cocoa Powder
- Simply Organic Vanilla
- Allergen Free Chocolate / Chocolate Chips
- Bob's Red Mill Pancake Mix
- Simple Mills Pizza Dough

Easy-ish Chocolate Chip Ice Cream Sandwiches

Ice cream of your choice

Chocolate chips cookies

½ cup of melted refined coconut oil or ½ cup melted
    butter

1 tsp vanilla

1 large egg

½ tsp baking powder

¼ tsp baking soda

½ tsp salt

2 cups of 1to1 gf flour

1 cup organic raw sugar

1 cup (or more) allergen-free semi-sweet chocolate chips

Directions:

- Preheat Oven to 375.

- Add wet ingredients to bowl and mix together, then
  add dry ingredients.

- Mix ingredients together with a hand mixer, spoon,
  or in a kitchen aid mixer.

- Spoon dough onto a baking sheet in an even number and keep space between the cookies.

- Bake for 10-12 minutes.

- Take out and, after a couple of minutes, transfer to a cooling rack and leave for 5 minutes. Then, place the cookies in the freezer for 30 minutes.

- After 30 minutes are up, take out cookies and ice cream. Scoop out ice cream onto one cookie and top with a second cookie to create the sandwich.

- Repeat until all cookies have been used.

- Eat immediately, or you can store them in the freezer until you're ready.

Appliances / Gadgets

- Kitchen Aid Mixer (we use this almost every day)

- Rice Cooker

- Juicer

- Crock Pot

- Can Opener (we rarely use this one, so you can get a hand crank one and save money)

- Bread maker

- Ninja Blender/Food Processor

Pans / Bakeware (no Teflon or nonstick)

- Stainless Steel

- Cast Iron

- Ceramic

- Glass

Easy-ish Blank Shopping List

Fruits and Vegetables

Seafood

Beef / Chicken

Baking Supplies

Dairy

Eggs

Bread

Snacks

Paper Supplies

Cleaning Supplies

Pet Items

Specialty items

Easy-ish Weekly Menu Tips and Tricks

- Plan your meals around what fruits and vegetables are in season. They will taste better and cost less.

- Ask your family to help with meal planning. I usually pose the question in our family group text while I'm working on our menu for the upcoming week.

- Make enough for dinner to have leftovers for lunch the next day.

- Prep on weekends when you have the time and get your kids involved. Our kids have been cooking in our kitchen since they were steady enough to stand on a chair and follow simple directions.

- You don't have to cook a complicated meal with a bajillion steps to have a fantastic dinner. Simple meals with good ingredients and seasonings are always a winner.

- It's faster to cook dinner or reheat leftovers for lunch than drive to a fast-food place. It's also better for your wallet and your health.

- You do not have to eat 100% "the right way" all the time. You are human, and you will be in situations where you won't be able to, or you just have a craving. We eat anti-inflammatory foods about 90+% of the time, and our son eats this way 95-98% of the time. So don't stress.

- You don't have to shop at Whole Foods, Trader Joe's, or that crazy expensive Erewhon grocery store. I do most of my shopping at Publix / Wegmans and then fill in with Amazon and Sprouts. Find a store that fits your needs and price points, then fill in with subscription services and specialty stores as needed.

- Shopping at the same store each week means you get to know the managers, and it's how you can ask them to carry a specific brand so you don't have to shop at their competitors instead, and they start regularly carrying it. (True story, y'all)

- Do move or switch your meals around to accommodate your schedule. Some meals are faster to make than others, even when you're keeping it easy-ish.

Easy-ish Sample Weekly Menu

Monday:

Breakfast – eggs, Van's gf waffles, and / or protein shake

Lunch – leftovers

Dinner – chicken empanadas with black beans and rice

Tuesday:

Breakfast – cassava-flour soft tortillas with eggs and
cheese

Lunch – empanadas with black beans and rice

Dinner – spaghetti and meatballs (make an extra pan of
meatballs to save for subs)

Wednesday:

Breakfast – eggs and / or protein shake

Lunch – leftover spaghetti and meatballs

Dinner – baked salmon, rice, and roasted green beans

Thursday:

Breakfast – eggs and / or protein shake

Lunch – leftover salmon, rice, and roasted green beans

Dinner – meatball subs (use meatballs from Tuesday) with carrots and cucumbers and homemade ranch dipping sauce

Friday:

Breakfast – eggs and / or protein shake

Lunch – leftover meatball subs

Dinner – chicken stir fry with rice and noodles

Saturday:

Breakfast – Van's gf waffles and eggs

Lunch – leftover chicken stir fry

Dinner – hamburgers on the grill with french fries and fruit

Sunday:

Breakfast – pancakes and eggs

Lunch – leftover hamburgers

Dinner – grilled chicken, baked potatoes, and collard greens

Easy-ish Blank Weekly Menu

Monday:

Breakfast –

Lunch –

Dinner –

Tuesday:

Breakfast –

Lunch –

Dinner –

Wednesday:

Breakfast –

Lunch –

Dinner –

Thursday:

Breakfast –

Lunch –

Dinner –

Friday:

Breakfast –

Lunch –

Dinner –

Saturday:

Breakfast –

Lunch –

Dinner –

Sunday:

Breakfast –

Lunch –

Dinner –

More Easy-ish Recipes

I'm not sharing super fancy recipes with y'all because I'm not a professional cook. (I don't really know how much of each seasoning I use, so I started with a minimum amount.) What I am sharing is how to take recipes that most of us love to eat and make them as anti-inflammatory as possible.

If you're like me, you don't want any kid (or adult) to be left out at parties or social events due to food allergies or dietary requirements, so these recipes can be modified to fit any requirement, except maybe vegan.

While there are vegan meat alternatives, the majority of them are filled with seed oils and chemicals that do your body no good and, frankly, in my opinion, do the opposite of what people who eat vegan are hoping to achieve with their health. Lastly, we cannot be plant-based since a plant-based diet would make our son's body work too hard to digest his food, and for him, lead to more inflammation.

Copy Cat Chick-fil-a
(Our Son's Favorite)

(I made several iterations of this recipe from different food bloggers until I developed one with modifications that fit our dietary needs and still tasted amazingly.)

¾ cup of dye-free pickle juice

¾ cup of milk (almond or cow)

3 eggs

2 pounds of boneless, skinless chicken thighs or chicken breasts cubed

Combine the above ingredients and marinate for at least an hour in the fridge. You can also prep the night before and marinate overnight!

3 cups of almond flour or gluten-free flour

1-2 tablespoons of paprika

2 teaspoons of powdered sugar (optional)

1 tablespoon of black pepper

1 tablespoon of salt

1 small bowl of one of the following: start with ½ cup of refined coconut oil (must be melted), olive oil, or avocado oil, and add as needed

Directions:

- Preheat Oven to 375
- Line baking pan with parchment paper
- Mix flour mixture together (add additional flour, spices, etc., as needed)
- Take marinated chicken from the fridge and drain
- Dredge the chicken in the flour mixture, then coat it with the oil of your choice by dipping it into the bowl, and then place it on the baking pan. Repeat until the chicken is gone or the pan is filled.
- Bake for 18 minutes, depending on your oven, and let cool.

Fettuccine Alfredo with Chicken (Our Daughter's Favorite)

1 boneless, skinless chicken breast or boneless, skinless chicken thigh per person, chopped into medium-sized chunks

2 cups of heavy whipping cream

1 ½ cups of parmesan cheese

2 tablespoons of unsalted butter

Salt and black pepper

GF Egg noodles or GF fettuccini noodles

Directions:

- Boil noodles according to instructions.
- While water is heating, cook chicken in a pan or cast iron skillet.
- Remove the chicken, but leave droppings, and cover the chicken to keep warm.
- Add heavy whipping cream, parmesan cheese, and unsalted butter to the pan, stir until blended and

butter has melted, then simmer for about 10 minutes (occasionally stirring).

- Add salt and black pepper to taste the sauce while simmering.

- Drain noodles.

- After 10 minutes, add noodles and chicken and mix them together.

- Enjoy!

- Double this recipe for leftovers while you cook, and you can enjoy this for lunch. Be sure to add a little water to it when you heat it up the next day.

Chicken Stir Fry
(Family Favorite)

1 boneless, skinless chicken breast or boneless, skinless chicken thighs, chopped into medium-sized chunks

1 cup of carrots (washed and peeled)

An entire container or bag of spinach (wash first)

1 bunch of bok choy (wash this several times first)

1 egg per person

2 cups of rice (Use your rice cooker. This can be prepared the day before and stored in the fridge, and always rinse your rice a few times before cooking it.)

1-2 tablespoons of olive oil or refined coconut oil

Seasonings:

Salt

Pepper

Ginger

Diced garlic or garlic powder

Onion Powder

Coconut Aminos

Directions:

- Use a wok or a large pan and pour in oil over medium heat.

- Start with the vegetables first to make sure they are cooked through. I season each round of cooking with the seasonings listed.

- Make a circle in the center and drop in eggs (add more oil if needed), then scramble and add seasonings.

- Remove eggs and vegetables, add more oil if needed, then add in chicken, seasonings, and coconut aminos. Cook until done (internal temp 165).

- Remove chicken and add to egg and vegetable mixture.

- Heat the rice if it is cold; if not, you can keep the chicken in the pan and add rice, egg, and vegetables, then stir together.

- Enjoy!

Meatball Subs
(Family Favorite)

1-2 lbs. of ground beef

mozzarella cheese

parmesan cheese

salt

pepper

oregano

onion powder

garlic powder

1-2 eggs

½ cup of almond flour

Sub rolls—we like to use Cristal Bread's Brand

Sauce:

1 small container of plain tomato sauce

salt

pepper

oregano

onion powder

garlic powder

Directions:

- Preheat Oven to 375

- Mix in seasonings (however much of each you like), eggs, and almond flour with the ground beef.

- Roll them into medium-sized meatballs (keep them as close to the same size as possible for even cooking) and place them on a baking sheet.

- Bake for about 25 minutes or until done.

- While the meatballs are baking, prepare your sauce by pouring plain tomato sauce into a saucepan and adding the seasonings—start with 1 tsp each and add to taste. Warm on medium heat until bubbles form, then turn down to low heat. Don't forget to stir.

- Optional: toast sub rolls

- After placing meatballs on sub rolls, add sauce, then cheese.

- Optional: Place meatball subs in the oven to melt cheese

- Enjoy!

Strawberry Shortcake Muffins with Homemade Whipped Cream

2 cups of almond flour

1 tsp of salt

1 tsp of baking soda

1 tsp of baking powder

½ cup of sugar

2 eggs

1 tsp of vanilla

½ cup of olive oil

½ cup of water

½ cup of almond milk

½ cup of maple syrup

Directions:

- Preheat oven to 325

- Combine ingredients for muffins together in one bowl and mix well.

- Pour mixture into muffin pan, about halfway for each muffin.
- Bake for about 18-20 minutes or until golden brown on top.
- Let cool for about five minutes.
- Add toppings.
- This will make twelve large muffins.

While the muffins are baking:

Toppings:

½ c to 1 cup of Strawberries

Directions:

- Wash
- Cut off tops
- Diced into large or small chunks (whatever you prefer)
- Set to the side in a bowl

Whipped Cream:

1 carton of heavy whipping cream

1 tsp of vanilla

1 tablespoon of honey

Directions:

- Pour into kitchen aid bowl or use a handheld mixer
- Whip until peaks form.
- Don't over-whip, or you'll end up with honey-vanilla butter

Closing Thoughts

With all these suggested changes, I wouldn't toss everything out at once because everything costs too freaking much at the time of writing this guide, and it's super overwhelming.

The most important changes you can make are the big three: oil, flour, and sugar. After that, I would replace items as they run out.

Also, you might have noticed that I don't list coffee, creamers, or even a coffee machine. My family and I don't drink coffee, no matter how sweet or creamed it is. It's just a taste preference, so find what works for you under the guidelines of good, anti-inflammatory ingredients!

Resources

Podcasts
Culture Apothecary with Alex Clark
Relatable with Allie Beth Stuckey
Office Ladies

Websites
TaylorDukesWellness
JovialFoods
TheFoodBabe
Be Well By Kelly
A Modern Homestead
Good Ranchers
White Oak Pastures
Let Them Eat Gluten Free Cake

About the Author

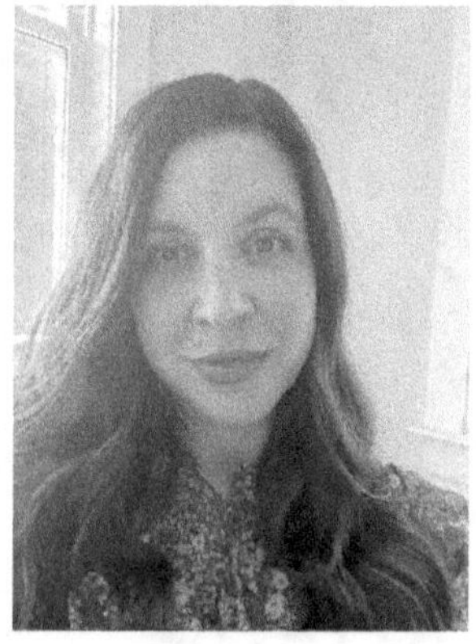

Marquita Valentine is a NYT and USA Today Bestselling author of contemporary romance. She is married to her high school sweetheart and lives on a farm near a small town in the south. To keep up with her latest releases, updated content, and sales, sign up for her newsletter by emailing her at marquita@marquita valentine.com.